Home Remedies

Powerful and Effective Natural Remedies to Cure Common Ailments Fast and Easy

Contents

Chapter 1. What are Herbal Remedies?

If you are looking for an alternative to medicine, either prescription or over the counter, you'll find that herbal remedies, also known as herbal recipes, are an alternative. They may be what you're looking for, and they're actually easy to use. Herbs have been used for medicine since ancient times, and these herbs have all been tried and proven over the course of time.

Sadly, many people will dismiss herbal recipes before they even try them out to see if they work. There are some herbs that will affect some people more strongly than others, and always make sure you aren't allergic to anything that you'd be using. It's a type of alternative medicine that almost eight percent of the world practices.

Clinical studies are being done to prove why these herbs help us with common and uncommon ailments, but the test of time has really already proven that the herbs work. There are many reasons that people decide to try out herbal medicine and recipes instead of just sticking to over the count or prescription solutions.

So Why Choose Herbal Recipes?

One of the main reasons that people decide to use herbal recipes, like the ones listed in this book, is so that they can avoid harmful side effects. Medicine today is made up of herbs and chemicals, and the chemicals in your medicine can cause side effects that are sometimes worse than what you're trying to cure. This is one of the main reasons that people choose herbs because they have little to no side effects at all.

You also have more options than just a pill, and sometimes herbal recipes actually taste good. Of course, remember that some herbs cannot be taken when you're pregnant, and you can't give a child under one year of age honey or you can put them in harm's way. Other than that, herbal recipes are extremely safe to use, and even children can use them, but often they have to be diluted for children that have yet to hit puberty.

Where Do You Get the Herbs?

There are many options for getting your herbs when you're looking to use herbal recipes to help cure common ailments. Often, you can go to a local health and food store and get everything you need, and some of the basic teas can be found in the local supermarket as well. If you're looking for raw honey, it can be found in supermarkets and health stores. If you're looking for local honey, you can go to a farmer's market, and the price is usually reasonable.

Of course, if you can't find something, many people will turn to the internet to get what they need. Just make sure that you're getting it from a respectable person who has good reviews and quality products. Look into who you're buying from, and make sure that the purity is there, especially when dealing with essential oils or extracts that you may be using for your herbal recipes. They should also advertise how fresh each batch of herbs they sell is, and that'll help you to know the potency of the herb you're getting, since potency fades over time.

Chapter 2. Cold & Flu Treatment Recipes

Being a viral, you can't really get rid of the cold or the flu, but you can treat the symptoms and boost your immune system so that you're sick for much less time overall. With the symptoms being taken care of, you'll feel that much better, feeling more like yourself. There are many herbal remedies that are easy to use, and these natural cures are safe to use. You don't have to worry about reactions in the same manner that you would need to if you were getting over the counter drugs, making the process of feeling better that much safer.

Recipe #1 Grand Ginger Tea

It's a simple recipe that only takes a few ingredients, and it'll only take a few minutes to make. When you're sick, it's great to have ginger on hand.

Ingredients:

1. 1 Cup Water
2. 2 Teaspoons Honey
3. 1 Teaspoon Lemon
4. 1 Inch Piece Ginger

Directions:

1. Put the hot water on the stove to boil or in a tea kettle to do the same thing. Many people will even microwave the water if you don't want to wait too long.
2. Make sure you peel your ginger so it'll get into the water, making your tea.
3. Finely grate the ginger root, putting it into the pot of hot water. Turn it off, and

let it simmer. If it gets cold before it's as strong as you want it to be, just turn the water on to simmer again.

4. While it's hot, mix in the two teaspoons of honey and lemon.

Recipe #2 The Raw Spoon of Health

If you're having a hard time with your throat, then you're going to want to try this recipe. It'll help you to boost your immune system, sooth your throat, and kill bacteria that may be causing or at least contributing to your illness.

Ingredients:

1. ½ Teaspoon Raw Coconut Oil
2. ½ Teaspoon Cinnamon, Ground
3. 1 Teaspoon Raw Honey

Directions:

1. Just mix all of the ingredients together into a spoon.

2. Eat it, and you should notice a difference in your sore throat almost immediately. It's recommended to take at least twice daily, but it won't hurt if you choose to do it more often.

Recipe #3 Medical Lemonade

If you like lemonade and honey, then you're likely to actually enjoy this natural cold and flu recipe. It's easy to make, and it actually tastes pretty good. You can take it as much as you like, but it's recommended to have once in the morning and once before you go to bed until symptoms improve.

Ingredients:

1. 1 Cup Water, Chilled

2. 2-3 Tablespoons Raw Honey

3. 5 Teaspoons Lemon Juice, Fresh

Directions:

1. This recipe is as simple to make as adding everything together. Make sure to whisk it together until you can't see the honey anymore. This will help to make it a little sweeter. Some people will add lime juice if it's still too bitter.
2. If you are having a hard time getting the lemon juice or honey to mix, you can heat it up slightly and mix it that way, which will be easier.
3. Drink up, and you should notice affects after one or two uses.

Recipe #4 The Power Puncher

This is an herbal recipe that is sure to knock out your cold and flu after just a few uses, and you'll be feeling better in no time. Of course, most people don't like the taste, but it has a lot of useful ingredients that are sure to help.

Ingredients:

1. 2 Teaspoons Ground ginger
2. 1 Clove Garlic, Chopped
3. ½ Teaspoon Cayenne Powder
4. 1 Green Tea Bag
5. 2 Teaspoons Honey
6. 1 Teaspoon Thyme
7. 1 Cup Water

Directions:

1. Start like you would with any tea, making sure to boil the water.
2. Next, put the garlic, thyme, ginger, cayenne powder and green tea bag into the water to steep. Loose leaf green tea will also work if you have it.

3. Then, make sure to strain everything out before you continue, putting honey in it to finish.

4. Drink at least two to three times daily for fast results.

Recipe #5 Garlic Flavored Lemonade

This is once again, sadly, a recipe that will help you to knock out your cold and flu, but it won't taste good unless you have strange taste buds. You'll need fresh lemon and garlic for the best results.

Ingredients:

1. 3 Cloves Garlic, Chopped
2. 2 Teaspoons Grated Ginger
3. 3 Tablespoons Honey
4. 1 Quart Water
5. 2 Fresh Lemons, Squeezed

Directions:

1. Grate your fresh ginger if it's not already grated, and make sure to mince three cloves garlic. Add it into the quart of water.
2. Let it steep for twenty minutes before adding the juice of two fresh lemons and the honey. Add more honey as you see fit.
3. Let steep for thirty minutes, and then strain the mixture to make it easier to drink.
4. Pour and drink at least twice daily. You should drink at least six to eight ounces each time.

Why These Ingredients?

There are many reasons to use these recipes, and the biggest reason is they actually work. Of course, it's proven because of the ingredients you are using. Garlic is an antibiotic and an herbal antiviral. Honey is known to soothe your throat and it is antiseptic, antimicrobial, and antibacterial. Lemon is high in vitamin C, which will help to strengthen your immune system and it'll kill off bacteria in your throat to help speed the healing process.

Cayenne powder is a stimulant and it'll help to prevent you from getting sicker. Thyme is also an herbal antibacterial and antiviral. Coconut oil is also known to sooth the throat and boost your immune system while cinnamon will help to spike your metabolism and start your body. It's an antifungal and antibacterial. Every ingredient in these recipes is made to help you fight the cold and flu fast, helping you to feel better only a few uses.

Chapter 3. Herbs to Help with Arthritis

You should never take your freedom of movement for granted because anyone who suffers from arthritis knows that with a small ailment it all can be taken away. There's no need to use expensive and potentially dangerous medications when you have natural herbal recipes to help you overcome your arthritis. Each ingredient is picked carefully, and it's all about fast results to help soothe your arthritis quickly and effectively.

Recipe #6 Simple Arthritis Tea

A simple tea is usually best, but it doesn't work as quickly as some slaves. It can help you, and the tea below isn't known to be hard to take or taste too badly. You can always add honey to taste, and some people use sugar. However, the sugar can be bad for you for a variety of reasons, and honey is recommended. Make sure you use raw honey so that it has all of its natural benefits.

Ingredients:

1. 2 Cups Water
2. 1 Teaspoon Grated Ginger
3. 1 Teaspoon Ground Turmeric
4. 2 Teaspoons Honey

Directions:

1. Make sure o boil the water, and then add grated ginger and the turmeric. Stir until all of the turmeric is dissolved.
2. Next, make sure to reduce it to simmer so that the ginger will get into the water to make your tea.

3. Turn the heat off, adding the honey and whisking until it is completely dissolved.

4. Let cool slightly, and drink at least once daily. It is recommended you do so during the morning, as it is known to produce the best results.

Recipe #7 A Molasses Shot

This is easy to take, but if you don't like the taste of blackstrap molasses, it will be hard to take. You need very few ingredients, and it takes very little time to take it every morning to get the best results. Just remember that it often has a laxative effect, and therefore it should not be taken more than once daily.

Ingredients:

1. 2 Tablespoons Warm Water

2. 1 Tablespoon Blackstrap Molasses

3. ½ Teaspoon Cinnamon

1. Mix everything together. Make sure the water is warm so that it dissolves the molasses that much easier.
2. Stir until it is a little less thick so that you can drink it. You may have to use a spoon or add more water.
3. Make sure to take it at least once daily to help with your arthritis and joint pain.

Recipe #8 Arthritis Berry Tea

These aren't just any berries if you want your arthritis to get better, and instead it needs to be juniper berries. You should never drink juniper berry tea when you're pregnant, and honey is optional but usually desired to keep this tea from being too bitter. Fresh juniper berries are hard to find, but luckily dried juniper berries will work best to make this tea.

Ingredients:

1.   2 Teaspoons Raw Honey
2.   1 Cup Water
3.   1 Tablespoon Dried Juniper Berries
4.   ½ Teaspoon Turmeric

Directions:

1.   Heat up the water like you would normal tea, adding the juniper berries and turmeric once it comes to a boil.
2.   Next, you need to let it steep for at least five to ten minutes to make a strong tea.
3.   Then, you need to strain it out and add honey while it's still warm, stirring until it's completely dissolved.
4.   Drink at least once daily, but not more than twice daily.

Recipe #9 A Helpful Oil Blend

Sometimes, a tea just won't cut it. Sometimes, you need something to rub on your joints for instant relief from your arthritis pain, and that's exactly what this recipe is meant to give you. For more instant results, this oil is best, and you can even make it in advance.

Ingredients:

1. 7 Drops Peppermint Oil
2. 2 Teaspoons Olive Oil
3. 6 Drops Eucalyptus Oil

Directions:

1. Just mix all of the oils together, and remember that your olive oil is your carrier oil.
2. Apply it to the affected area, and you should notice results in about five to ten minutes. Add more as needed throughout the day.

Why These Ingredients?

From your teas which offer more long term relief to the oil that you can rub into your skin, offering immediate relief, each of these ingredients are needed. Make sure to never skip a corner if you want arthritis relief. Peppermint and eucalyptus oil have pain relieving effects, and the cooling sensation help your discomfort. Sadly, these oils won't help in the long term. Blackstrap molasses has magnesium, calcium, and potassium, which is great for arthritis.

You have to use it at least once daily for a while to get quick results. Honey is a natural sweetener, and has a real effect on arthritis pain due to anti-inflammatory properties. However, olive oil is actually anti-inflammatory when rubbed into your joints. Turmeric and ginger are known as anti-inflammatories, as well as juniper berries. It'll help to reduce inflammation pain. You should also keep in mind that cinnamon can be added to help with the oil as well, but it can be taken internally, such as in the tea described above. Cinnamon is also an anti-inflammatory, helping to get rid of your arthritis pain in the long and short term depending on how it is used.

Chapter 4. Treating High Blood Pressure

If you suffer from high blood pressure, you've probably already tried many different medications with horrible side effects or no results. Talk to your doctor about any of the herbal recipes below to help you control your high blood pressure in a natural manner, helping you to limit the side affects you experience while lowering your high blood pressure in a steady and healthy manner. Just remember that like with most high blood pressure remedies, including medication, you'll need to wait for effects. They will not be immediate.

Recipe #10 A Coconut Blast

Blast your high blood pressure away by making sure that you

Ingredients:

1. 1 Cup Coconut Water
2. 2 Teaspoons Cinnamon
3. 1 Teaspoon Honey

Directions:

1. Start by just making sure that all ingredients are mixed together. Try to get the cinnamon thoroughly mixed with the honey first, as it'll make it that much easier.
2. Then drink it chilled two to three times daily to help lower your blood pressure over time.

Recipe #11 Chocolate Hibiscus Tea

This isn't exactly a tea, but it is made very similarly to one. You'll enjoy the taste, as it's both earthy and sweet. You'll be able to drink it at least once daily to help you lower your blood pressure, and each ingredient is picked out carefully to make sure you get the best results.

Ingredients:

1. ½ Teaspoon Cinnamon
2. 1 Cup Water
3. 1 Teaspoon Honey
4. 2 Teaspoons Raw Cocoa Powder
5. 3 Teaspoons Dried Hibiscus

Directions:

1. Start by boiling the water so that you can make your tea.
2. Once the water has started to boil, you can turn it to a simmer and place in the

hibiscus. Let it simmer while stirring for about two to three minutes.

3. Strain the hibiscus out, and then add in the honey, cinnamon, and cocoa powder.

4. Pout into a cup and drink either hot or chilled about once daily.

Recipe #12 A Red Smoothie

If you're looking for something with a little more flavor, you can try this red smoothie once a day to help you lower your high blood pressure over time. It's even tasty, and you can always add an extra fruit into the mix if you want to, making it a little sweeter.

Ingredients:

1. ½ Cup Ice

2. ¼ Cup Beet Juice

3. 2 Teaspoons Cinnamon

4. 4 Teaspoons Honey

5. ½ Cup Pomegranate Juice

Directions:

1. Start by making sure your blender is clean, and blend together the ice and juices. Make sure that it is thoroughly blended.
2. Then, make sure to add the honey and cinnamon, stirring until it's mixed all the way through.
3. Drink this once a day, and the best results are found when it's taken in the morning.

Recipe #13 A Red Morning Shot

If you're used to taking a shot, you'll be able to take this powerful packed shot in the morning to get through your day and lower your blood pressure over time. Of course, you'll find that it may not taste very good. You can always dilute it with more water, but because the taste isn't desired it's not recommended.

Ingredients:

1. 1 Teaspoon Cinnamon
2. 4 Ounces Cranberry Juice
3. ½ Teaspoon Garlic Powder
4. 1 Teaspoon Oregano

Directions:

1. Making the Red Morning Shot is pretty easy, and all you have to do is mix everything together.
2. Down it as quickly as you can unless you just like the taste. Do this twice daily if you want stronger results.

Recipe #14 The Mild & Sweet Fix

This is a fix if your blood pressure isn't too high yet. It has a relatively pleasant taste, making it easy to take on a regular basis. It isn't even hard to fix, and it can help to prevent high blood pressure as well.

Ingredients:

1. 1 Cup Chilled Hibiscus Tea
2. ½ Cup Pomegranate Juice
3. 2 Teaspoons Honey

Directions:

1. Just mix it all together, making sure the honey is completely dissolved in the drink mixture or it'll settle to the bottom.
2. Drink it at least once a day, but you can drink it more often if you like.

Why These Ingredients?

Coconut water is used because it increases muscle function, and the heart is a muscle. It's meant to help your heart become stronger and lower your blood pressure in the process. It has potassium and magnesium. Not only does cinnamon help you to lower blood pressure, but it will also help you to control your blood sugar levels as well. Honey is antioxidant rich, and therefore can help promote heart health when put into these recipes as well.

Hibiscus is commonly used because it has also been proven to lower high blood pressure in human studies. It contains bioactive phytochemicals which will help you with your high blood pressure because it's like an ACE inhibitor. Cocoa powder will also help you if no sugar is added because the flavonols that can be found in raw cocoa will help you to relax your blood vessels, and it also thins your blood.

Beet juice is great for high blood pressure because it's a source of potassium as well as folate. These are great ways to regulate your high blood pressure, and pomegranate juice is useful because it also acts an ACE inhibitor, keeping your blood vessels from constricting as much, releasing the pressure. Cranberry juice is yet another wonderful way to control your blood pressure because it an antioxidant and anti-inflammatory, which helps to reduce any damage to your blood vessels, in turn lowering your blood pressure.

As far as herbs go, garlic is also important to lowering blood pressure. Of course, fresh is always best, as it has anti-hypertension properties. Oregano is another unlikely aid to your quest for lowering high blood pressure because it contains carvacrol which is a compound which has been linked to lowering the heart rate and therefore your high blood pressure.

Chapter 5. Curing Your Acne

Acne is more than just a problem. It's actually an embarrassment, but once again there is no reason for you to have to buy expensive medications, over the counter or prescription. There are many natural recipes that you can use with the right herbs to help you to make sure that your acne is gotten rid of fast. Some recipes offer quicker results, but remember to continue using whichever one you choose for a few days even after it seems the acne has disappeared if you want to keep it gone.

Recipe #15 A Simple Aloe Solution

You can grow aloe vera all on your own, and that's the best way to get the most potent aloe for your acne. Just cut open the plant, and you'll be able to get the gel directly from the middle of the stem, also commonly referred to as an aloe leaf. Of course, you can also buy aloe gel on the market. Try to get it as pure as you can.

Ingredients:

1. 2 Teaspoons Aloe Vera Gel
2. 2-3 Drops Tea Tree Oil

Directions:

1. Put your aloe gel in something where you can mix in the few drops of tea tree oil.
2. Wash the affected area, patting it dry. Then, apply the mixture onto it. Let it sit on it as it soaks into your skin. There is no need to wash it off.

3. Do this two to three times daily for quick results. You can make it up in advance for up to three or five days if placed in an airtight container in the fridge.

Recipe #16 A Liquid Applications

These herbs are great to help you get rid of your acne fast, and you can wash your face about thirty minutes afterwards for the best results. You need to let the ingredients work their magic for as long as possible, and you can make it up in advance. Once again, it should be put in an airtight container and only made up three to four days in advance.

Ingredients:

1. 2 Teaspoons Fresh Lemon Juice
2. 5-6 Drops Tea Tree Oil
3. 2 Teaspoons Water
4. ¼ Cup Green Tea

Directions:

1. Just mix all of the ingredients together in a bowl.
2. Make sure to use a cotton ball for application. Dip it into the mixture, getting it damp.
3. Apply it to the affected area. If you are reusing the mixture, never dip the cotton ball into it twice. Do this two to three times daily if you want your acne gone fast.

Recipe #17 A Very Green Wash

This is yet another facial wash which will require you to have cotton balls on hand for its application. Follow the same rules when making it up in advance, and try to use it three to four times daily.

Ingredients:

1. ½ Cup Cool Green Tea
2. 1 Teaspoon Aloe Vera Gel
3. 1 Teaspoon Honey
4. 6-7 Drops Mint Oil

Directions:

1. Mix everything together. You may have to heat up the green tea to dissolve the honey, but chill it again before using.
2. Apply using a cotton ball to the affected area. Let it sit there for at least fifteen to twenty minutes.
3. Wash the area gently, and pat dry.

Recipe #18 The Simplistic Facemask

Sometimes when acne is being very stubborn, you'll need to have more than a wash or a liquid application. This is where a facemask is best, as you can let it sit and work on the area for a little while. It doesn't matter when you put it on, but do it at least once every other day.

Ingredients:

1. 4 Tablespoons Honey
2. 2 Teaspoons Apple Cider Vinegar
3. 5-6 Drops Basil Oil

Directions:

1. Make sure that you add everything together. It should be mixed all the way through.
2. Apply a thick layer to the affected area, and let it sit for twenty minutes.
3. Wash it off afterwards with cool water. Make sure you pat the area dry so you don't make it break open. Apply at least twice a day, usually morning and night.

Why These Ingredients?

Every herb listed is chosen for a particular reason, and it's all meant to help you get rid of your acne as quickly as you can without the use of harsh chemicals. Tea tree oil will help to fight any inflammation you're experiencing due to your acne, which also makes acne worse. Aloe has soothing properties as well as cleansing ones, and it also has anti-inflammatory properties, allowing your pores to open and be cleansed.

Make sure that when you're using lemon juice, you're using it fresh. It can be helpful in treating acne because of its acidic nature, as it'll help to clean out dirt. Green tea can be made in advance, but don't sweeten it with honey. This is why you shouldn't buy it premade. Green tea contains many antioxidants, which helps to fight acne. Its best when it's used after it's been cooled in the fridge.

Honey is a sticky solution to acne, but it is a solution because of its antibiotic properties. Mint oil is a soothing solution, making it a very popular herbal recipe. It'll help to remove oil that is clogging your pores, and you can even make your own mint oil if you diffuse it after growing your own.

Apple cider vinegar should always have the mother in it, which you'll find in organic or raw apple cider vinegar, and it's extremely helpful when curing acne. It exfoliates your skin, and it's also known to reduce red marks. Of course, you should never forget basil oil, as it's an herb that helps because it has antibacterial and anti-inflammatory aspects, helping to get rid of your acne quickly and effectively. There are many combinations to use, but the recipes above are sure to help you cure your acne breakouts in a reasonable time.

Chapter 6. Helping with Seasonal Allergies

Seasonal allergies can be a plague, and they make you feel downright miserable. Often, allergy medications don't do the trick, and herbal remedies and recipes will work better. Not all of these recipes will work immediately, but you'll notice an effect over time, and some are meant to help you with symptoms fast.

Recipe #19 The Citrus Twister

This is a great drink that you can take, and you don't have to worry about it tasting bad. It's always best if an herbal recipe also tastes great or is easy to use, as you're more likely to use it on a regular basis. To get the best results, try to drink it at least once daily, but twice daily is better.

Ingredients:

1. 2 Teaspoons Lemon Juice
2. 2 Teaspoons Honey
3. 4 Teaspoons Ice Water
4. ¼ Cup Fresh Orange Juice

Directions:

1. Squeeze your juice fresh if you want the best results, and then mix in the honey until it's dissolved.
2. Add in the water, and stir again.
3. Chill for at least an hour, and then drink once or twice daily.

Recipe #20 The Quick Cleanser

This is a recipe that is meant to help provide relief from your symptoms quickly, and therefore it's not known for its taste. Luckily, it's pretty easy to make and use. You can even take it like a shot.

Ingredients:

1. 1 Teaspoon Raw Apple Cider Vinegar
2. ½ Teaspoon Raw Honey
3. 1 Teaspoon Fresh Lemon Juice
4. ½ Teaspoon Turmeric
5. ½ Teaspoon Water

Directions:

1. You can just mix everything together like you would a shot, but don't expect it to look appetizing.
2. Take it quickly, and some people like to wash it down with something that has a strong and delightful taste, helping it to

be a little more tolerable. Try it at least once daily.

Recipe #21 A Turmeric Tumbler

This is yet another wonderful remedy that has turmeric in it, helping to provide you with relief as a decongestant almost immediately. Luckily, this one is known to taste a little better, and you can take it more than once daily.

Ingredients:

1. 2 Teaspoons Turmeric
2. 1 ½ Teaspoons Local Honey
3. 1 Cup Fresh Orange Juice
4. ½ Teaspoon Gingko Powder

Directions:

1. Fresh orange juice will help to cover up the taste of the herbs while providing

you the vitamin C that you need. Just mix it all together.

2. Try to get it mixed thoroughly, as it'll make it taste a little better.

3. Make sure it's chilled and down it or sip it. Just make sure to take it at a minimum once daily.

Recipe #22 A Tablespoon of Helpfulness

This is just one tablespoon, so like the taste or not, you'll be able to deal with it if it'll help you to get relief from your allergies. It's easy to make, and you can even keep minced garlic on hand to make the process a little easier. Take it each and every morning if you want results. Some people take it three times daily.

Ingredients:

1. 1 Teaspoon Raw, Local Honey
2. ½ Teaspoon Minced Garlic

3. ½ Teaspoon Ginger

Directions:

1. Mix it all into one large tablespoon and
    take it.
2. Wash it down with water if it sticks in
    your mouth, but remember it has to be
    taken once daily at a minimum.

Recipe #23 Ginger & Lemon Tea

If you're looking for just a tea that you can drink to help suppress allergies, look no further. This simple to make ginger tea will help you to take care of your allergies so long as you take it on a regular basis. Taking it at around the same time will help to increase the results, helping you a little more. The nettle leaves are also a help, but you won't taste them all that much since they don't have a strong flavor.

Ingredients:

1. 2 Teaspoons Grated Ginger, Fresh
2. 1 ½ Teaspoons Lemon Juice, Fresh
3. 1 Cup Water
4. 2 Teaspoons Honey
5. 2 Tablespoons Dried Nettle Leaves

Directions:

1. Heat up the water like you would for normal tea.
2. Add in the ginger and nettle leaves, allowing it to steep to taste. The stronger, the better.
3. Strain the herbs out, and then add the honey and lemon juice to drink it.

Why These Ingredients?

Vitamin C will help boost your immune system, which will help you to deal with seasonal allergies by providing relief. Make sure to boost your immune system regularly, and orange juice and lemon juice is sure to do it. Honey is also great for allergy relief, but only if it's raw and organic. Local honey is usually best because it has small traces of pollen from your area, helping you to build a tolerance when consumed regularly.

When facing seasonal allergies, it is usually best to have a decongestant on your side, which is exactly what both apple cider vinegar and turmeric are. Apple cider vinegar is also able to help cut down on mucus production as a whole, helping to keep your nasal passages clear for a while to come.

Gingko is a powder that you can find in most local health and food stores, and you can sometimes find it at an herbal pharmacy. It is great at relieving allergy symptoms, and that's because it's anti-inflammatory properties providing relief within twenty to thirty minutes.

Garlic may not be everyone's favorite herbal remedy, but it's easy to grow and easy to use. Better yet, it's an herbal antibiotic, helping to ward off infection. Not only will it fight your seasonal allergies, but it'll help to prevent sinus infections as well. The antioxidants help as well.

Ginger is also known to help suppress any allergic reaction you may be experiencing, as well as being anti-inflammatory and containing a lot of antioxidants. Of course, don't forget nettle leaves which are a natural antihistamine, helping to stop your seasonal allergies in their tracks, keeping you healthy throughout the allergy season.

Chapter 7. Treating Harmful Nausea

It doesn't matter if you're experiencing normal nausea or morning sickness. These herbal remedies will stop it in its tracks, and they're all made to be fast acting. Many of them can be taken on the onset of nausea, but they'll work if you let it go until it gets bad as well, in case you can't get anywhere to make them. They're quick and easy to make too.

Recipe #24 Peppermint & Ginger Tea

Ginger is known to help you get rid of nausea quickly, but peppermint is soothing as well. When you mix the two together, you're sure to find a relief from your nausea quickly. Many people actually experience relief almost immediately with this nausea remedy, but it's not as quick to make as other natural recipes.

Ingredients:

1. 2 Tablespoons Grated Ginger, Fresh
2. 3 Teaspoons Dried Peppermint Leaves
3. 1 Cup Water
4. 2 Teaspoons Honey

Directions:

1. Start by boiling water, like you would for any tea. Of course, if you want it to boil faster, it will only take a few minutes in the microwave.
2. Next, let the ginger and peppermint leaves steep. If you don't have peppermint leaves, peppermint extract or oil is also known to work.
3. Strain all of the herbs out, adding the honey to taste. You can always add more

or less as needed. Take it as soon as you feel nausea coming on.

Recipe #25 Clove & Ginger Tea

Teas are usually the best thing when you're trying to fight nausea, and ginger is one of the best and well proven methods to help with nausea. You can pair it with a lot of other helpful herbs when you want to help with nausea, and clove is one of those wonderful herbs to pair it with.

Ingredients:

1. 1 Teaspoons Grated Clove
2. 2 Teaspoons Grated Ginger, Fresh
3. 1 ½ Teaspoons Honey
4. 1 Teaspoon Lemon Juice, Fresh

Directions:

1. Make the tea normally, making sure to strain out all of the herbs after three to five minutes. If the tea is stronger, it'll help, but make sure that it stays warm.
2. Add in the lemon juice and honey at the same time. Make sure it's dissolved before drinking. You can drink it whenever you have nausea.

Recipe #26 Just a Tablespoon

If you're looking for nausea relief without a tea because you want something a little quicker, than this recipe is best. However, it's not as potent as the teas. You can take it while you're waiting on a tea to clear up the rest of it as well, though.

Ingredients:

1. 1 Tablespoon Honey
2. 1 Teaspoon Lemon Juice, Fresh

1. To get rid of nausea in just minutes, mix the honey and lemon juice together.
2. Make sure that you take it slowly, licking it off the spoon. If you take it too quickly, then you might upset your stomach more. The honey helps to balance out the acidity.

Recipe #27 Another Quick Tablespoon

Again, you may not be able to wait for a tea to brew if you're feeling that bad. It's good to have a few options that you can just throw together, and this is one of them, making it easier to get rid of your nausea than ever.

Ingredients:

1. ½ Teaspoon Cinnamon
2. 1 Tablespoon Honey

3. ½ Teaspoon Ground Ginger

Directions:

1. Mix everything together. Try to make sure there are no clumps in the powder so it's easier to take.
2. Just eat it slowly so that you can get rid of your nausea quickly.

Recipe #28 Mint & Lemon Water

This isn't a tablespoon of anything, and instead it's actually a drink. However, it doesn't have to be prepared like tea will, making it another quick and easy solution. There is no reason that you should have to deal with nausea any longer than you have to. Many people will add honey to the mixture to sweeten it, but it's not necessary.

Ingredients:

1. 1 Cup Water, Chilled
2. 2 Teaspoon Lemon Juice
3. ½ Teaspoon Peppermint Extract

Directions:

1. Having the water chilled makes it a little easier to drink for many people. So just

    mix the lemon juice and peppermint extract together.

2. Take it whenever you feel nauseous, helping you to get rid of it without much hassle. Sipping at it usually helps the most because you aren't rushing your stomach with it, but you're stimulating your digestive system in a slow but steady manner. It's important you get rid of whatever is causing you to feel ill as quick as possible if you want to be free of nausea for some time to come instead of just temporarily.

Why These Ingredients?

You can use powdered ginger if you don't have it fresh, but you'll get the best results with fresh ginger on hand. Ginger is known to help with nausea because it promotes digestive juices to help you calm your stomach down and move the process along. Clove is great at curing nausea, but it can also help if you have cold or even a runny nose. It doesn't matter if it's powdered or just the clove oil, but it's helpful because it's an antiviral and antifungal.

Of course, lemon juice will also help with morning sickness. It's even safe to take during pregnancy. Honey is a wonderful home remedy for almost everything, and it'll help to calm your stomach too as well as sooth any sore throat you may be having.

What most people don't know is that cinnamon can help you to get rid of your nausea as well, and it's sitting right in your spice cabinet. However, it's not good to use it when you're pregnant. Cinnamon will help to stimulate your digestive system, helping you to get rid of nausea and what's causing it quickly.

Chapter 8. Fixing Stomach Aches Fast

Just like nausea, there is no reason to try to deal with a stomachache when there are natural recipes that you can try to help you get rid of it. Often, it's just a few simple ingredients that you already have laying around. Take a leap and try any of these herbal recipes to get rid of your stomachache without the use of processed medication.

Recipe #29 Chamomile & Lemon Tea

If you're looking for a quick fix, this is a tea that is soothing, but be careful because it can help you sleep as well. It'll help you to feel better within five to ten minutes. For some people it does take up to twenty, but not for many. Often, you'll see results fast.

Ingredients:

1. 2 Teaspoons Dried Chamomile
2. 1 Teaspoon Honey
3. 1 ½ Teaspoons Fresh Lemon Juice
4. 1 Cup Water

Directions:

1. Make this tea like any other, and make sure to get out every bit of herbs to make drinking it a little easier.
2. Add the honey into the water, and stir in the fresh lemon juice once the herbs are strained out. It won't hurt you to take this remedy more than once a day.

Recipe #30 Peppermint & Honey Drink

This isn't a tea, and it's much easier to make, helping you to make it quicker in case of severe pain. A severe stomachache isn't something you want to wait to fix, so just keep the water cold and you're ready to use this remedy anytime you want to fix your stomachache fast.

Ingredients:

1. 1 Cup Water, Chilled
2. 1 Teaspoon Peppermint Extract
3. 2 Teaspoons Honey

Directions:

1. Mix everything together until all of the honey is dissolved. The smell of peppermint will also help you to soothe your stomach.
2. Sip at the drink, and do not just down it or you may upset your stomach further instead of helping it.

Recipe #31 Something to Eat

You can actually help your stomachache by eating something, and it doesn't even taste that bad if you like the taste of licorice. Many people say that fennel tastes similarly, which is what you'll be eating to help you get rid of your stomach upset.

Ingredients:

1. ½ Teaspoon Fennel Seeds
2. 1 Tablespoon Honey

Directions:

1. Just mix them together, and eat it slowly. You'll need to chew the fennel seed up.
2. Take it whenever you feel the onset of stomachaches, as it'll work a little better.

Recipe #32 Lime Water with a Twist

If you're looking for something to help quickly without making a tea once again, t hen you'll find this is yet another recipe that is easy to make. Just keep the ingredients on hand and the water chilled, and it'll be an easy fix to any stomach pain you're experiencing.

Ingredients:

1. ½ Teaspoon Peppermint Extract
2. 2 Teaspoons Lime Juice
3. 1 Teaspoon Honey
4. 1 Cup Water, Chilled

Directions:

1. This is great if you don't like lemon because it's a little too sharp, and the honey helps to even it out a little as well. Mix all of your ingredients together.

2. Everything should be completely mixed into the water, and then you can sip at it. Some people even like it over ice.

Recipe #33 A Soothing Cold Drink

Cold drinks are great when you're experiencing stomach pain, and this herbal recipe is no different. It is great for that extremely bad stomach pain, as it is fast acting and packs a powerful punch. It can help with many of the symptoms immediately, giving you relief fast.

Ingredients:

1. ½ Cup Chilled Aloe Vera Juice
2. ½ Cup Chilled Water
3. 1 Teaspoon Honey
4. ½ Teaspoon Peppermint Extract
5. ½ Teaspoon Apple Cider Vinegar

Directions:

1. Make sure to mix the apple cider vinegar and the water first. Then add in the aloe juice, making sure it doesn't have added sugars.
2. Add in the peppermint extract and honey at the same time, mixing well.
3. Sip at the drink slowly, and you'll notice relief comes quickly.

Recipe #34 The Simple & Quick Fix

If you need something quick and simple to make because you just aren't feeling well, then try this recipe. There's almost nothing to it, but it'll make a big difference in helping you feel better sooner.

Ingredients:

1. 1 Cup Chilled Aloe Vera Juice
2. 2 Teaspoons Lemon Juice

Directions:

1. Just mix it together and drink it slowly. It's really that easy. You can even make it advance or right on the spot. It sits in the fridge just fine.
2. If it's not sweet enough, add honey or a little less lemon juice.

Why These Ingredients?

Chamomile is known to soothe you when your stomach is aching. It'll also help you to reduce your stress, which may be causing the stomach pain in the first place. Chamomile will help the bloating that you're feeling from stomach pain. Lemon can also help you to soothe your stomach, and it can be added to almost any tea to give it that added effect. Lemon juice will also work, but fresh lemon juice is always best because it aids the digestive process that much better. Honey promotes rehydration of the body, which can help you to get rid of your stomach pain.

Fennel seed is often chewed to help with stomachaches because it improves digestion, and it can also eliminate bloating. Since it eliminates bloating, you'll feel some relief within just five minutes most of the time. Lime is like lemon, helping to stimulate the digestive process, and it's used in place of lemon a lot if you think lemon is too sour to use.

Aloe juice is great if you're trying to get rid of harsh stomach pain, and that's because it treats bloating, constipation, as well as diarrhea, which may be causing your stomach pain in the first place. You can also use apple cider vinegar because it stimulates digestive juices.

Chapter 9. Recipes for Headaches & Migraines

Most headaches are from pain, anxiety, and tension. Of course, there are many ways to get rid of a headache with herbal recipes, so there are many options before you. You'll find that they all work quickly to provide you the relief that you're desperately in need of. So make sure that you use one of them next time you have a migraine or headache issue so that you can avoid harsh and processed medicines when a natural solution is available.

Recipe #35 The Cayenne Crusher

This may not sound like it'll actually work, but cayenne is great for headaches. It's not the most pleasant herbal remedy if you can't handle spice, but if you're spice fanatic it's best. It'll also help you to relieve your headache or migraine quickly.

Ingredients:

1. 3 Ounces Warm Water
2. 1 Teaspoon Powdered Cayenne Pepper

Directions:

1. This is one of the simplest headache recipes that you can make because all you do is mix it together, making sure nothing settles at the bottom.
2. Down it quickly because sipping at it will only build up the heat.

Recipe #36 A Feverfew Tea

It may seem strange because feverfew is most commonly known to treat fever, but it's also a quick way to get rid of a really bad headache or migraine. This tea is easy to make, and you can sweeten it with honey since it's never good to add sugar on top of a headache.

Ingredients:

1. 2 Teaspoons Dried Feverfew
2. 1 Cup Water
3. 2 Teaspoons Honey

Directions:

1. Just make the tea like you normally would, allowing it to come to a boil and then steep.
2. Strain out all of the herbs, and then add honey. Drink slowly, and you should notice relief within fifteen to thirty minutes depending on how strong you made your tea.

Recipe #37 A Cold Drink for Relief

If you want to drink something cold and still have something that will help you to relieve your headache or even the worst migraine, then this is the herbal recipe for you. It's easy to make, and you can make it in advance if you have chronic migraines.

Ingredients:

1.   1 Teaspoon Peppermint Extract
2.   1 Cup Chilled Water
3.   1 Teaspoon Ginger

Directions:

1.   Just mix everything together, and it's really that easy to have a drink that will help you to relieve your headaches.
2.   Just make sure it's cold and diffused properly. Fresh ginger is usually best,

but if you use fresh ginger then you'll need to grate it and let it sit in the water for at least an hour before straining and adding the peppermint extract.

Recipe #38 Oils to the Rescue

You'll find that sometimes you can get rid of a headache by applying a few oils topically as well, including peppermint oil. Of course, for this oil combination you will need a carrier oil, as rosemary oil is very potent. In this recipe your carrier oil is olive oil, and it'll even help to moisturize your skin, but olive oil does not directly affect your headache.

Ingredients:

1. 1 Tablespoon Olive Oil
2. 2-3 Drops Rosemary Oil
3. 2-3 Drops Peppermint Oil

Directions:

1. Mix all of your oils together, making sure that it is done thoroughly.
2. Lightly apply it to your temples, rubbing it in a circular pattern. Apply this at the onset of a headache or migraine for the best results.

Recipes #39 A Lavender & Rosemary Rub

Another topical oil you can use has lavender, and it only takes a few moments for it to work. It's one of the quickest ways to help make sure that you get rid of your headache or migraine pain almost immediately. Some people find it helps in as little as three to five minutes. If you don't feel an effect, just apply it again, as an extra dose will usually do the trick.

Ingredients:

1.   3-4 Drops Lavender Oil
2.   2-3 Drops Rosemary Oil
3.   ½ Teaspoon Olive Oil

Directions:

1.   Mix all of your oils together before applying to your temples.

2. Rub in small circles on your temples to help relieve the pressure and tension fast. The faster it's relieved, the sooner you'll start to feel relief from this oil mixture. Try to lay in a dark room and calm your mind if the headache is too bad, as it'll help the remedy to work a little faster.

Why These Ingredients?

Cayenne pepper is known to treat pain, and it's an anti-inflammatory as well, making it the perfect headache solution. The best part is that it's known to work quickly as well. Feverfew is a great tea to use because it helps to relax the blood vessels in your head, helping to reduce some of the worst headaches, including a migraine. If you catch it early enough, you can knock it out with feverfew entirely sometimes.

Peppermint is once again a very useful herbal extract to keep around because it can help you to release the tension that may be causing your migraine, as it promotes relaxation. Of course, ginger is also able to help with a headache, especially if it is a sinus related headache or migraine.

Rosemary oil is also a great oil to use when you're trying to get rid of a headache or migraine with a topical solution. It is therapeutic when you apply it and inhale it, and it can produce a tingling sensation that helps to release tension. It's commonly used with peppermint oil for the best results.

You can also use lavender topically to help you get rid of any migraine or headache that you may be having. You always need to apply it with a carrier oil, and if you react too strongly to it,

you can always add a little more of your carrier
oil on top of the applied batch, such as olive oil.

Chapter 10. Herbal Help for Anxiety

When you're stressed or anxious, you really need to find something to help. Being anxious or stressed out will affect your health, including causing weight gain, depression, and even disrupting your sleep which will spiral out over time to cause even more health problems. From oils to teas, there are way to naturally control your stress and anxiety, and you can use most of these recipes fairly often, keeping your anxiety levels completely manageable.

Recipe #40 The Simplest Oil Rub

For something simple and quick that you can do every day, it's sometimes best to just have something that you can apply to your temples.

Some people can handle lavender oil on its own, but a carrier oil is sometimes best. You don't even need a lot to help you with your anxiety, and it can even stave off anxiety attacks if used early enough.

Ingredients:

1. ½ Teaspoon Olive Oil
2. 3-5 Drops Lavender Oil

Directions:

1. Remember that purity matters with your lavender oil, and you'll be able to mix it directly with the carrier oil, applying it to your temples.
2. If you feel the need, just rub it into your temples gently to release the anxiety right away.

Recipe #41 A Helpful Tea

This tea wont' make your drowsy, making it a great way to naturally handle your anxiety, so don't worry. Instead, just make the tea and try to relax. It will help a little less if you are trying to do stressful activities while you're enjoying the tea that you've made.

Ingredients:

1. ½ Teaspoon Dried Lemon Balm
2. 1 Teaspoon Green Tea Leaves
3. 2 Teaspoons Honey
4. 1 Cup Water

1. Make it like you normally would for just about any tea, and let it simmer for at least five minutes. Always keep in mind that if the tea is stronger, then it'll be more likely to help because the potency is a little stronger.

2. Add honey to taste, so make sure to add more or less if you like, but only do so after straining the herbs out.

3. Drink slowly, and drink warm. A warm drink is also known to help with anxiety.

Recipe #42 A Passionflower Tea

This is another tea that you can use when you're having issues with anxiety. Try to hit anxiety off before it builds too high, becoming too much for you to handle. Natural remedies and recipes will work better if you act quickly when you feel anxiety coming on, and you can even use most of these teas, including this one, as a preventative measure. Anxiety builds up, and you probably have tension from anxiety before you even notice it. Be careful, though, as passion flower can actually make you sleepy.

Ingredients:

1. 2 Teaspoons Honey, Raw
2. 1 Cup Water
3. 1 Teaspoon Dried Passionflower
4. ½ Teaspoon Dried Lemon Balm

Directions:

1. Again, this tea will need to be made like normal. The passionflower shouldn't make you sleepy, making it perfect for just about any time of the day.
2. Add the honey when you have everything strained out, and remember that hot

drinks help more than cold ones, but you can still ice it if you desire too. It'll hurt even less to ice it if you're using it as a preventative measure to keep your anxiety levels down.

Recipe #43 Lavender & Passionflower Tea

This is yet another mixture that is going to help make sure that you reduce your anxiety, but it can make you very sleepy. It's best to use if your anxiety is keeping you up at night, so be careful not to take it when you have somewhere to go. These herbs are great at releasing tension and stress quickly, and they've withstood the test of time. You can get dried lavender rather easily, as well.

Ingredients:

1. 2 Teaspoons Lavender, Dried

2. 1 Teaspoon Passionflower, Dried

3. 2 Teaspoons Honey

4. 1 Cup Water

5. ½ Teaspoon Dried Licorice Root

Directions:

1. Start by making it like you would normal tea, and add in the licorice root, passionflower, and lavender too steep for as long as you want, but keep it hot.

2. Then strain, adding the honey to taste. Drink warm, and you'll be relaxed and off to sleep in no time, able to wake up fresh and anxiety free.

Why These Ingredients?

Lavender oil is easy to use, and it's great even if you just use the lavender in tea form. It's an anti-anxiety herb that will help to relax tension, and it is great when used as a type of aromatherapy when applied to the temples where most of your stress is usually seen.

Green tea is also helpful if you are trying to minimize your anxiety, and it works relatively quickly as well, helping you to get over anxiety quickly. You'll find that green tea has L-theanine, which will help to stop a rising heart rate as well as rising blood pressure. It helps you to calm yourself, and it's easy to use. Honey is also known to help because it'll help to boost you r immune system and therefore mental health. This makes you less likely to feel the effects of anxiety as strongly.

Passionflower is a tea that you can find commonly, and if you can't find the dried herb, you can always just get premade passionflower tea, since it's common to find at any supermarket. Passionflower is a sedative, so make sure to only use it before bed. Licorice root is also known to help with any anxiety that you may be experiencing, and you don't even have to use that much of it to get fast results. It contains a natural hormone, which will allow your body to handle stressful situations a little better. It's an alternative to cortisone, and it's a great way to calm your mind. It

Chapter 11. What to Keep in Mind

One of the biggest parts about learning to use herbal recipes is learning how to store your herbs so that they stay good and that their potency stays good as well. Using top herbs is going to affect how your herbal recipes come out, and if they're to potent enough, you may find that the herbal recipe doesn't work at all.

This is why fresh ingredients usually work best when you're trying to get quick results. Of course, some herbs are just easier to us when dried, and it's easier to get dried herbs overall. Storing them become simple when you know the rules, but make sure that you have everything labeled properly, as many dried herbs look the same unless you really know what to look for, and you don't want to grab the wrong one when you're in a pinch.

As a rule of thumb, it is best to replace your herbs every six months to a year, but keep fresh ingredients on hand as well. You don't have to throw away honey. Even if honey crystalizes so long as it is raw honey, you can heat it back up and it'll be just fine. Any local honey is raw honey so long as there has been no added sugar.

How to Store Herbs:

You need to make sure that you have airtight containers. Mason jars are usually recommended because you can clearly see the herbs, and moisture won't get through. You'll even be able to label by writing on the mason jars, the lids, or putting a piece of tape on it and writing on that. This will help you with the labeling process. A screw cap is known to keep out moisture best, which is another reason that mason jars are usually recommended.

You need to store herbs in a cool and dry location as well. Of course, herbs also need to be out of the light. Light can affect your herbs, so if you do use mason jars, try to get tinted ones or at least make sure that they are foggy to help keep the sunlight out. It's usually best to store them in a cabinet or pantry, where there are no windows to let light in that will ruin your herbs.

How to Make it Cost Effective:

Many people are hesitant to try herbal recipes because it isn't cost effective to store or buy them. However, there are many of these herbs that you can grow and dry yourself, and it's as easy as growing them in a pot. There's little work to growing herbs, and you can buy in bulk to make sure that you have all of the containers you need. usually your best deal with come from a craft store sale, repurposing glass containers like baby food jars, or getting them online. If you're careful, you can usually get cheap herbs online as well if you're buying them in bulk, but don't get too large of a bulk or your herbs will go bad before you use them.